RECIPE INDEX

PAGE #	RECIPE NAME

MEAL PLAN

MONDAY

TUESDAY

WEDNESDAY

THURSDAY

FRIDAY

SATURDAY

SUNDAY

SHOPPING LIST

Recipe For

_____

Ingredients

Instructions

Recipe For

_____

Ingredients

___ _____
___ _____
___ _____
___ _____
___ _____
___ _____
___ _____
___ _____
___ _____
___ _____
___ _____
___ _____

Instructions

_____
_____
_____
_____
_____
_____
_____
_____
_____
_____
_____
_____

Recipe For

_____

Ingredients

Instructions

Recipe For

_____

Ingredients

_____	_____
_____	_____
_____	_____
_____	_____
_____	_____
_____	_____
_____	_____
_____	_____
_____	_____
_____	_____
_____	_____

Instructions

_____
_____
_____
_____
_____
_____
_____
_____
_____
_____
_____

Recipe For

_____

Ingredients

Instructions

Recipe For

_____

Ingredients

____	_____
____	_____
____	_____
____	_____
____	_____
____	_____
____	_____
____	_____
____	_____
____	_____
____	_____

Instructions

_____
_____
_____
_____
_____
_____
_____
_____
_____
_____

Recipe For

_____

Ingredients

____	_____
____	_____
____	_____
____	_____
____	_____
____	_____
____	_____
____	_____
____	_____
____	_____
____	_____

Instructions

_____
_____
_____
_____
_____
_____
_____
_____
_____
_____
_____

MEAL PLAN

MONDAY

TUESDAY

WEDNESDAY

THURSDAY

FRIDAY

SATURDAY

SUNDAY

SHOPPING LIST

Recipe For

_____

Ingredients

Instructions

Recipe For

_____

Ingredients

_____	_____
_____	_____
_____	_____
_____	_____
_____	_____
_____	_____
_____	_____
_____	_____
_____	_____
_____	_____
_____	_____
_____	_____

Instructions

_____
_____
_____
_____
_____
_____
_____
_____
_____
_____
_____
_____

Recipe For

_____

Ingredients

_____
_____
_____
_____
_____
_____
_____
_____
_____
_____
_____

Instructions

_____
_____
_____
_____
_____
_____
_____
_____
_____
_____

Recipe For

_____

Ingredients

___ _____
___ _____
___ _____
___ _____
___ _____
___ _____
___ _____
___ _____
___ _____
___ _____

Instructions

_____
_____
_____
_____
_____
_____
_____
_____
_____
_____
_____

Recipe For

_____

Ingredients

_____ _____
_____ _____
_____ _____
_____ _____
_____ _____
_____ _____
_____ _____
_____ _____
_____ _____
_____ _____
_____ _____

Instructions

_____
_____
_____
_____
_____
_____
_____
_____
_____
_____

Recipe For

_____

Ingredients

___	_____
___	_____
___	_____
___	_____
___	_____
___	_____
___	_____
___	_____
___	_____
___	_____
___	_____

Instructions

_____
_____
_____
_____
_____
_____
_____
_____
_____
_____

Recipe For

_____

Ingredients

Instructions

MEAL PLAN

MONDAY

TUESDAY

WEDNESDAY

THURSDAY

FRIDAY

SATURDAY

SUNDAY

SHOPPING LIST

Recipe For

_____

Ingredients

_____ _____
_____ _____
_____ _____
_____ _____
_____ _____
_____ _____
_____ _____
_____ _____
_____ _____
_____ _____

Instructions

_____
_____
_____
_____
_____
_____
_____
_____
_____
_____

Recipe For

_____

Ingredients

____ _____
____ _____
____ _____
____ _____
____ _____
____ _____
____ _____
____ _____
____ _____
____ _____
____ _____

Instructions

_____
_____
_____
_____
_____
_____
_____
_____
_____
_____
_____

Recipe For

_____

Ingredients

____	_____
____	_____
____	_____
____	_____
____	_____
____	_____
____	_____
____	_____
____	_____
____	_____
____	_____
____	_____

Instructions

_____
_____
_____
_____
_____
_____
_____
_____
_____
_____
_____

Recipe For

_____

Ingredients

_____
_____
_____
_____
_____
_____
_____
_____
_____
_____
_____

Instructions

_____
_____
_____
_____
_____
_____
_____
_____
_____
_____
_____

Recipe For

_____

Ingredients

_____
_____
_____
_____
_____
_____
_____
_____
_____
_____
_____

Instructions

_____
_____
_____
_____
_____
_____
_____
_____
_____
_____
_____

Recipe For

_____

Ingredients

___	_____
___	_____
___	_____
___	_____
___	_____
___	_____
___	_____
___	_____
___	_____
___	_____
___	_____

Instructions

_____
_____
_____
_____
_____
_____
_____
_____
_____
_____
_____

Recipe For

_____

Ingredients

_____
_____
_____
_____
_____
_____
_____
_____
_____
_____
_____

Instructions

_____
_____
_____
_____
_____
_____
_____
_____
_____
_____

MEAL PLAN

MONDAY

TUESDAY

WEDNESDAY

THURSDAY

FRIDAY

SATURDAY

SUNDAY

SHOPPING LIST

Recipe For

_____

Ingredients

_____	_____
_____	_____
_____	_____
_____	_____
_____	_____
_____	_____
_____	_____
_____	_____
_____	_____

Instructions

_____
_____
_____
_____
_____
_____
_____
_____
_____
_____

Recipe For

_____

Ingredients

____	_____
____	_____
____	_____
____	_____
____	_____
____	_____
____	_____
____	_____
____	_____
____	_____
____	_____
____	_____

Instructions

_____
_____
_____
_____
_____
_____
_____
_____
_____
_____
_____
_____

Recipe For

_____

Ingredients

_____

Instructions

_____

Recipe For

_____

Ingredients

Instructions

Recipe For

_____

Ingredients

_____
_____
_____
_____
_____
_____
_____
_____
_____
_____

Instructions

_____
_____
_____
_____
_____
_____
_____
_____
_____
_____
_____
_____

Recipe For

_____

Ingredients

_____ _____
_____ _____
_____ _____
_____ _____
_____ _____
_____ _____
_____ _____
_____ _____
_____ _____
_____ _____
_____ _____

Instructions

_____
_____
_____
_____
_____
_____
_____
_____
_____
_____
_____

Recipe For

_____

Ingredients

Instructions

MEAL PLAN

MONDAY

TUESDAY

WEDNESDAY

THURSDAY

FRIDAY

SATURDAY

SUNDAY

SHOPPING LIST

Recipe For

_____

Ingredients

_____ _____
_____ _____
_____ _____
_____ _____
_____ _____
_____ _____
_____ _____
_____ _____
_____ _____
_____ _____
_____ _____

Instructions

_____
_____
_____
_____
_____
_____
_____
_____
_____
_____
_____

Recipe For

_____

Ingredients

_____	_____
_____	_____
_____	_____
_____	_____
_____	_____
_____	_____
_____	_____
_____	_____
_____	_____
_____	_____

Instructions

_____
_____
_____
_____
_____
_____
_____
_____
_____
_____
_____

Recipe For

_____

Ingredients

___	_____
___	_____
___	_____
___	_____
___	_____
___	_____
___	_____
___	_____
___	_____
___	_____
___	_____

Instructions

_____
_____
_____
_____
_____
_____
_____
_____
_____
_____

Recipe For

_____

Ingredients

___	_____
___	_____
___	_____
___	_____
___	_____
___	_____
___	_____
___	_____
___	_____

Instructions

_____
_____
_____
_____
_____
_____
_____
_____
_____
_____
_____

Recipe For

_____

Ingredients

_____ _____
_____ _____
_____ _____
_____ _____
_____ _____
_____ _____
_____ _____
_____ _____
_____ _____
_____ _____
_____ _____
_____ _____

Instructions

_____
_____
_____
_____
_____
_____
_____
_____
_____
_____
_____

Recipe For

_____

Ingredients

_____

Instructions

_____

Recipe For

_____

Ingredients

Instructions

MEAL PLAN

MONDAY

TUESDAY

WEDNESDAY

THURSDAY

FRIDAY

SATURDAY

SUNDAY

SHOPPING LIST

Recipe For

_____

Ingredients

___	_____
___	_____
___	_____
___	_____
___	_____
___	_____
___	_____
___	_____
___	_____
___	_____
___	_____

Instructions

_____
_____
_____
_____
_____
_____
_____
_____
_____
_____

Recipe For

_____

Ingredients

_____ _____
_____ _____
_____ _____
_____ _____
_____ _____
_____ _____
_____ _____
_____ _____
_____ _____
_____ _____

Instructions

_____
_____
_____
_____
_____
_____
_____
_____
_____
_____

Recipe For

_____

Ingredients

Instructions

Recipe For

_____

Ingredients

_____	_____
_____	_____
_____	_____
_____	_____
_____	_____
_____	_____
_____	_____
_____	_____
_____	_____
_____	_____

Instructions

_____
_____
_____
_____
_____
_____
_____
_____
_____
_____

Recipe For

_____

Ingredients

_____ _____
_____ _____
_____ _____
_____ _____
_____ _____
_____ _____
_____ _____
_____ _____
_____ _____
_____ _____

Instructions

_____
_____
_____
_____
_____
_____
_____
_____
_____
_____
_____

Recipe For

_____

Ingredients

_____

_____

_____

_____

_____

_____

_____

_____

_____

_____

_____

_____

Instructions

_____

_____

_____

_____

_____

_____

_____

_____

_____

_____

Recipe For

_____

Ingredients

_____ _____
_____ _____
_____ _____
_____ _____
_____ _____
_____ _____
_____ _____
_____ _____
_____ _____
_____ _____
_____ _____
_____ _____

Instructions

_____
_____
_____
_____
_____
_____
_____
_____
_____
_____
_____

MEAL PLAN

MONDAY

TUESDAY

WEDNESDAY

THURSDAY

FRIDAY

SATURDAY

SUNDAY

SHOPPING LIST

Recipe For

_____

Ingredients

_____ _____
_____ _____
_____ _____
_____ _____
_____ _____
_____ _____
_____ _____
_____ _____
_____ _____
_____ _____

Instructions

_____
_____
_____
_____
_____
_____
_____
_____
_____
_____

Recipe For

_____

Ingredients

___	_____
___	_____
___	_____
___	_____
___	_____
___	_____
___	_____
___	_____
___	_____
___	_____
___	_____

Instructions

_____
_____
_____
_____
_____
_____
_____
_____
_____

Recipe For

_____

Ingredients

_____
_____
_____
_____
_____
_____
_____
_____
_____
_____
_____

Instructions

_____
_____
_____
_____
_____
_____
_____
_____
_____
_____

Recipe For

_____

Ingredients

_____
_____
_____
_____
_____
_____
_____
_____
_____
_____

Instructions

_____
_____
_____
_____
_____
_____
_____
_____
_____

Recipe For

_____

Ingredients

_____

_____

_____

_____

_____

_____

_____

_____

_____

_____

Instructions

_____

_____

_____

_____

_____

_____

_____

_____

_____

_____

_____

_____

Recipe For

_____

Ingredients

_____	_____
_____	_____
_____	_____
_____	_____
_____	_____
_____	_____
_____	_____
_____	_____
_____	_____
_____	_____
_____	_____
_____	_____

Instructions

_____
_____
_____
_____
_____
_____
_____
_____
_____
_____
_____
_____
_____

Recipe For

_____

Ingredients

___	_____
___	_____
___	_____
___	_____
___	_____
___	_____
___	_____
___	_____
___	_____
___	_____
___	_____

Instructions

_____
_____
_____
_____
_____
_____
_____
_____
_____
_____
_____

MEAL PLAN

MONDAY

TUESDAY

WEDNESDAY

THURSDAY

FRIDAY

SATURDAY

SUNDAY

SHOPPING LIST

Recipe For

_____

Ingredients

_____
_____
_____
_____
_____
_____
_____
_____
_____
_____

Instructions

_____
_____
_____
_____
_____
_____
_____
_____
_____

Recipe For

_____

Ingredients

___	_____
___	_____
___	_____
___	_____
___	_____
___	_____
___	_____
___	_____
___	_____
___	_____
___	_____

Instructions

_____
_____
_____
_____
_____
_____
_____
_____
_____
_____
_____

Recipe For

_____

Ingredients

___ _____
___ _____
___ _____
___ _____
___ _____
___ _____
___ _____
___ _____
___ _____
___ _____
___ _____
___ _____

Instructions

_____
_____
_____
_____
_____
_____
_____
_____
_____
_____
_____

Recipe For

_____

Ingredients

___	_____
___	_____
___	_____
___	_____
___	_____
___	_____
___	_____
___	_____
___	_____
___	_____

Instructions

_____
_____
_____
_____
_____
_____
_____
_____
_____
_____
_____

Recipe For

_____

Ingredients

____	_____
____	_____
____	_____
____	_____
____	_____
____	_____
____	_____
____	_____
____	_____
____	_____

Instructions

_____
_____
_____
_____
_____
_____
_____
_____
_____
_____
_____

Recipe For

_____

Ingredients

_____
_____
_____
_____
_____
_____
_____
_____
_____
_____
_____
_____

Instructions

_____
_____
_____
_____
_____
_____
_____
_____
_____
_____
_____

Recipe For

_____

Ingredients

_____ _____
_____ _____
_____ _____
_____ _____
_____ _____
_____ _____
_____ _____
_____ _____
_____ _____
_____ _____
_____ _____
_____ _____

Instructions

_____
_____
_____
_____
_____
_____
_____
_____
_____
_____
_____
_____
_____

MEAL PLAN

MONDAY

TUESDAY

WEDNESDAY

THURSDAY

FRIDAY

SATURDAY

SUNDAY

SHOPPING LIST

Recipe For

_____

Ingredients

___	_____
___	_____
___	_____
___	_____
___	_____
___	_____
___	_____
___	_____
___	_____
___	_____

Instructions

_____
_____
_____
_____
_____
_____
_____
_____
_____
_____

Recipe For

_____

Ingredients

___	_____
___	_____
___	_____
___	_____
___	_____
___	_____
___	_____
___	_____
___	_____
___	_____
___	_____

Instructions

_____
_____
_____
_____
_____
_____
_____
_____
_____
_____
_____
_____

Recipe For

_____

Ingredients

_____   _____
_____   _____
_____   _____
_____   _____
_____   _____
_____   _____
_____   _____
_____   _____
_____   _____
_____   _____

Instructions

_____
_____
_____
_____
_____
_____
_____
_____
_____
_____
_____

Recipe For

_____

Ingredients

___	_____
___	_____
___	_____
___	_____
___	_____
___	_____
___	_____
___	_____
___	_____
___	_____

Instructions

_____
_____
_____
_____
_____
_____
_____
_____
_____
_____
_____

Recipe For

_____

Ingredients

Instructions

Recipe For

_____

Ingredients

___	_____
___	_____
___	_____
___	_____
___	_____
___	_____
___	_____
___	_____

Instructions

_____
_____
_____
_____
_____
_____
_____
_____
_____
_____

Recipe For

_____

Ingredients

_____
_____
_____
_____
_____
_____
_____
_____
_____
_____
_____
_____
_____

Instructions

_____
_____
_____
_____
_____
_____
_____
_____
_____
_____
_____

MEAL PLAN

MONDAY

TUESDAY

WEDNESDAY

THURSDAY

FRIDAY

SATURDAY

SUNDAY

SHOPPING LIST

Recipe For

_____

Ingredients

___	_____
___	_____
___	_____
___	_____
___	_____
___	_____
___	_____
___	_____
___	_____
___	_____

Instructions

_____

_____

_____

_____

_____

_____

_____

_____

_____

_____

Recipe For

_____

Ingredients

_____
_____
_____
_____
_____
_____
_____
_____
_____
_____
_____
_____

Instructions

_____
_____
_____
_____
_____
_____
_____
_____
_____
_____
_____
_____

Recipe For

_____

Ingredients

____	_____
____	_____
____	_____
____	_____
____	_____
____	_____
____	_____
____	_____
____	_____
____	_____

Instructions

_____
_____
_____
_____
_____
_____
_____
_____
_____
_____
_____

Recipe For

_____

Ingredients

___	_____
___	_____
___	_____
___	_____
___	_____
___	_____
___	_____
___	_____
___	_____

Instructions

_____
_____
_____
_____
_____
_____
_____
_____
_____

Recipe For

_____

Ingredients

_____ _____
_____ _____
_____ _____
_____ _____
_____ _____
_____ _____
_____ _____
_____ _____
_____ _____

Instructions

_____
_____
_____
_____
_____
_____
_____
_____
_____

Recipe For

_____

Ingredients

Instructions

Recipe For

_____

Ingredients

Instructions

MEAL PLAN

MONDAY

TUESDAY

WEDNESDAY

THURSDAY

FRIDAY

SATURDAY

SUNDAY

SHOPPING LIST

Recipe For

_____

Ingredients

_____
_____
_____
_____
_____
_____
_____
_____
_____
_____
_____

Instructions

_____
_____
_____
_____
_____
_____
_____
_____
_____
_____
_____

Recipe For

_____

Ingredients

Instructions

Recipe For

_____

Ingredients

___	_____
___	_____
___	_____
___	_____
___	_____
___	_____
___	_____
___	_____
___	_____
___	_____

Instructions

_____
_____
_____
_____
_____
_____
_____
_____
_____
_____

Recipe For

_____

Ingredients

_____
_____
_____
_____
_____
_____
_____
_____
_____
_____
_____

Instructions

_____
_____
_____
_____
_____
_____
_____
_____
_____
_____
_____
_____

Recipe For

_____

Ingredients

_____ _____
_____ _____
_____ _____
_____ _____
_____ _____
_____ _____
_____ _____
_____ _____
_____ _____
_____ _____

Instructions

_____
_____
_____
_____
_____
_____
_____
_____
_____
_____
_____

Recipe For

_____

Ingredients

_____ _____
_____ _____
_____ _____
_____ _____
_____ _____
_____ _____
_____ _____
_____ _____
_____ _____
_____ _____
_____ _____
_____ _____

Instructions

_____
_____
_____
_____
_____
_____
_____
_____
_____
_____
_____

Recipe For

_____

Ingredients

_____ _____
_____ _____
_____ _____
_____ _____
_____ _____
_____ _____
_____ _____
_____ _____
_____ _____
_____ _____

Instructions

_____
_____
_____
_____
_____
_____
_____
_____
_____
_____

MEAL PLAN

MONDAY

TUESDAY

WEDNESDAY

THURSDAY

FRIDAY

SATURDAY

SUNDAY

SHOPPING LIST

Recipe For

_____

Ingredients

___	_____
___	_____
___	_____
___	_____
___	_____
___	_____
___	_____
___	_____
___	_____
___	_____
___	_____

Instructions

_____
_____
_____
_____
_____
_____
_____
_____
_____
_____

Recipe For

_____

Ingredients

_____   _____
_____   _____
_____   _____
_____   _____
_____   _____
_____   _____
_____   _____
_____   _____
_____   _____
_____   _____
_____   _____

Instructions

_____
_____
_____
_____
_____
_____
_____
_____
_____
_____
_____

Recipe For

_____

Ingredients

Instructions

Recipe For

_____

Ingredients

_____	_____
_____	_____
_____	_____
_____	_____
_____	_____
_____	_____
_____	_____
_____	_____
_____	_____
_____	_____
_____	_____

Instructions

_____
_____
_____
_____
_____
_____
_____
_____
_____
_____
_____
_____

Recipe For

_____

Ingredients

_____ _____
_____ _____
_____ _____
_____ _____
_____ _____
_____ _____
_____ _____
_____ _____
_____ _____

Instructions

_____
_____
_____
_____
_____
_____
_____
_____
_____
_____

Recipe For

_____

Ingredients

___	_____
___	_____
___	_____
___	_____
___	_____
___	_____
___	_____
___	_____
___	_____
___	_____
___	_____
___	_____
___	_____

Instructions

_____
_____
_____
_____
_____
_____
_____
_____
_____
_____
_____
_____

Recipe For

_____

Ingredients

___	_____
___	_____
___	_____
___	_____
___	_____
___	_____
___	_____
___	_____
___	_____
___	_____
___	_____

Instructions

_____
_____
_____
_____
_____
_____
_____
_____
_____

MEAL PLAN

MONDAY

TUESDAY

WEDNESDAY

THURSDAY

FRIDAY

SATURDAY

SUNDAY

Recipe For

_____

Ingredients

___	_____
___	_____
___	_____
___	_____
___	_____
___	_____
___	_____
___	_____
___	_____

Instructions

_____
_____
_____
_____
_____
_____
_____
_____
_____
_____

Recipe For

_____

Ingredients

_____
_____
_____
_____
_____
_____
_____
_____
_____
_____
_____
_____

Instructions

_____
_____
_____
_____
_____
_____
_____
_____
_____
_____

Recipe For

_____

Ingredients

_____	_____
_____	_____
_____	_____
_____	_____
_____	_____
_____	_____
_____	_____
_____	_____
_____	_____
_____	_____
_____	_____

Instructions

_____
_____
_____
_____
_____
_____
_____
_____
_____
_____
_____

Recipe For

_____

Ingredients

_____ _____
_____ _____
_____ _____
_____ _____
_____ _____
_____ _____
_____ _____
_____ _____
_____ _____
_____ _____
_____ _____

Instructions

_____
_____
_____
_____
_____
_____
_____
_____
_____
_____
_____
_____

Recipe For

_____

Ingredients

_____
_____
_____
_____
_____
_____
_____
_____
_____

Instructions

_____
_____
_____
_____
_____
_____
_____
_____
_____

Recipe For

_____

Ingredients

_____

Instructions

_____

Recipe For

_____

Ingredients

_____ _____
_____ _____
_____ _____
       _____
_____ _____
_____ _____
       _____
_____ _____
_____ _____
_____ _____
_____ _____

Instructions

_____
_____
_____
_____
_____
_____
_____
_____
_____
_____
_____

MEAL PLAN

MONDAY

TUESDAY

WEDNESDAY

THURSDAY

FRIDAY

SATURDAY

SUNDAY

SHOPPING LIST

Recipe For

_____

Ingredients

_____
_____
_____
_____
_____
_____
_____
_____
_____
_____

Instructions

_____
_____
_____
_____
_____
_____
_____
_____
_____
_____

Recipe For

_____

Ingredients

_____

Instructions

_____

Recipe For

_____

Ingredients

___ _____
___ _____
___ _____
___ _____
___ _____
___ _____
___ _____
___ _____
___ _____
___ _____

Instructions

_____
_____
_____
_____
_____
_____
_____
_____
_____

Recipe For

_____

Ingredients

_____
_____
_____
_____
_____
_____
_____
_____
_____

Instructions

_____
_____
_____
_____
_____
_____
_____
_____
_____

Recipe For

_____

Ingredients

_____ _____
_____ _____
_____ _____
_____ _____
_____ _____
_____ _____
_____ _____
_____ _____
_____ _____
_____ _____

Instructions

_____
_____
_____
_____
_____
_____
_____
_____
_____
_____

Recipe For

_____

Ingredients

Instructions

Recipe For

_____

Ingredients

_____	_____
_____	_____
_____	_____
_____	_____
_____	_____
_____	_____
_____	_____
_____	_____
_____	_____
_____	_____
_____	_____

Instructions

_____
_____
_____
_____
_____
_____
_____
_____
_____
_____
_____

MEAL PLAN

MONDAY

TUESDAY

WEDNESDAY

THURSDAY

FRIDAY

SATURDAY

SUNDAY

SHOPPING LIST

Recipe For

_____

Ingredients

_____ _____
_____ _____
_____ _____
_____ _____
_____ _____
_____ _____
_____ _____
_____ _____

Instructions

_____
_____
_____
_____
_____
_____
_____
_____
_____
_____

Recipe For

_____

Ingredients

___ _____
___ _____
___ _____
___ _____
___ _____
___ _____
___ _____
___ _____
___ _____
___ _____
___ _____

Instructions

_____
_____
_____
_____
_____
_____
_____
_____
_____
_____

Recipe For

_____

Ingredients

_____
_____
_____
_____
_____
_____
_____
_____
_____
_____
_____
_____

Instructions

_____
_____
_____
_____
_____
_____
_____
_____
_____
_____
_____
_____

Recipe For

_____

Ingredients

_____ _____
_____ _____
_____ _____
_____ _____
_____ _____
_____ _____
_____ _____
_____ _____
_____ _____
_____ _____

Instructions

_____
_____
_____
_____
_____
_____
_____
_____
_____
_____

Recipe For

_____

Ingredients

Instructions

Recipe For

_____

Ingredients

____	_____
____	_____
____	_____
____	_____
____	_____
____	_____
____	_____
____	_____
____	_____
____	_____
____	_____
____	_____

Instructions

_____
_____
_____
_____
_____
_____
_____
_____
_____
_____
_____
_____

Recipe For

_____

Ingredients

Instructions

www.ingramcontent.com/pod-product-compliance
Lightning Source LLC
Chambersburg PA
CBHW081552280526
45788CB00011B/3455